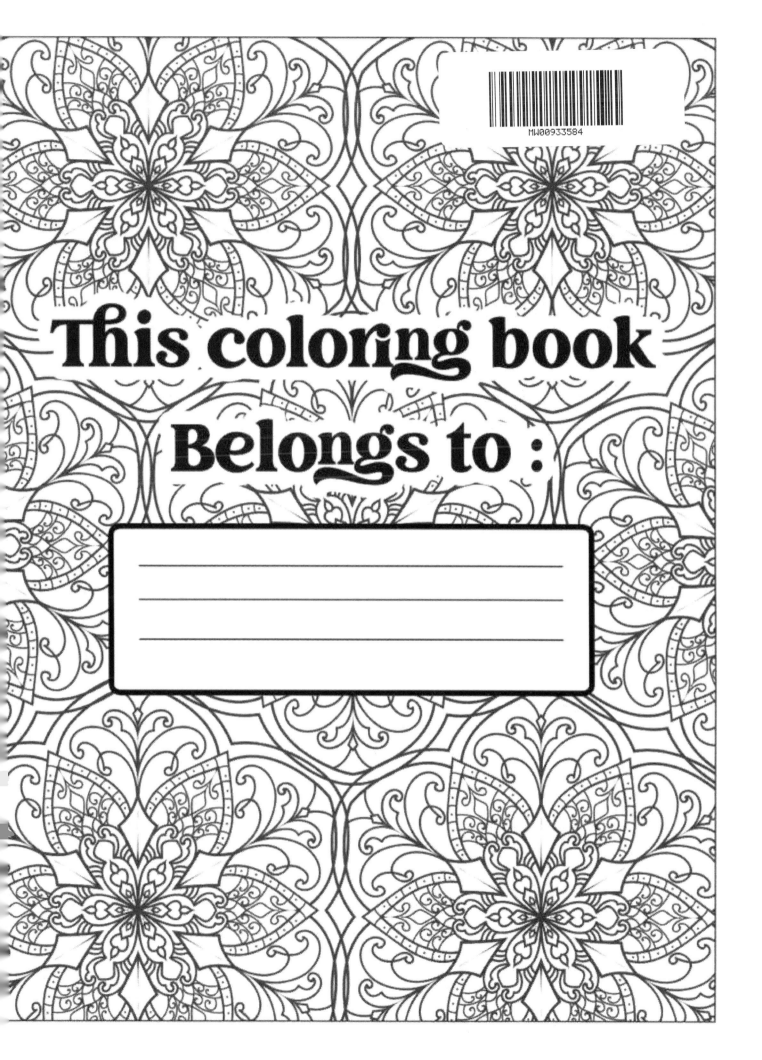

This coloring book
Belongs to :

COLOR TEST PAGE

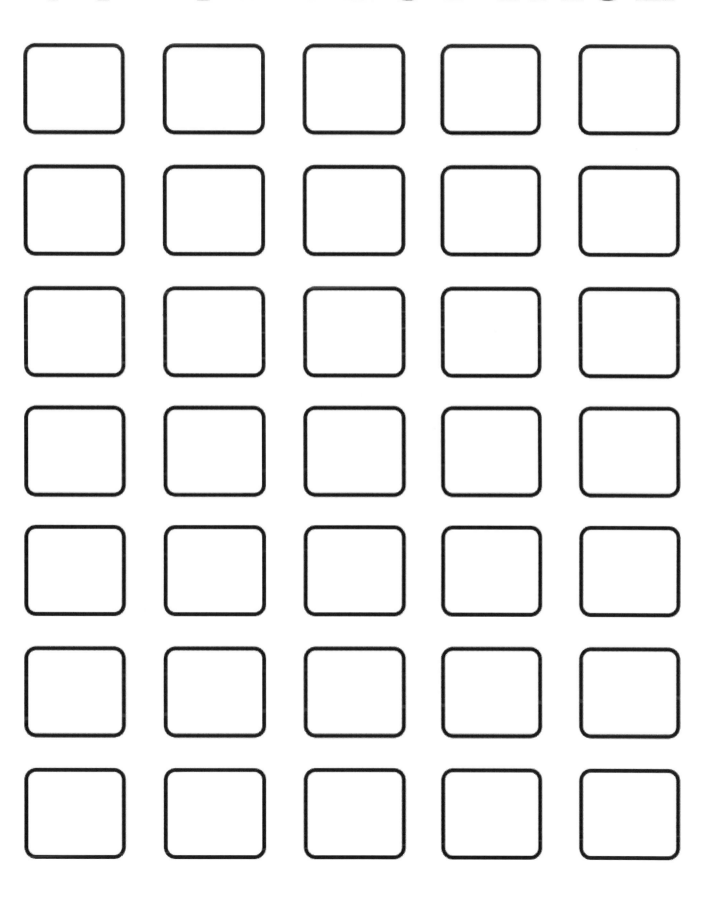

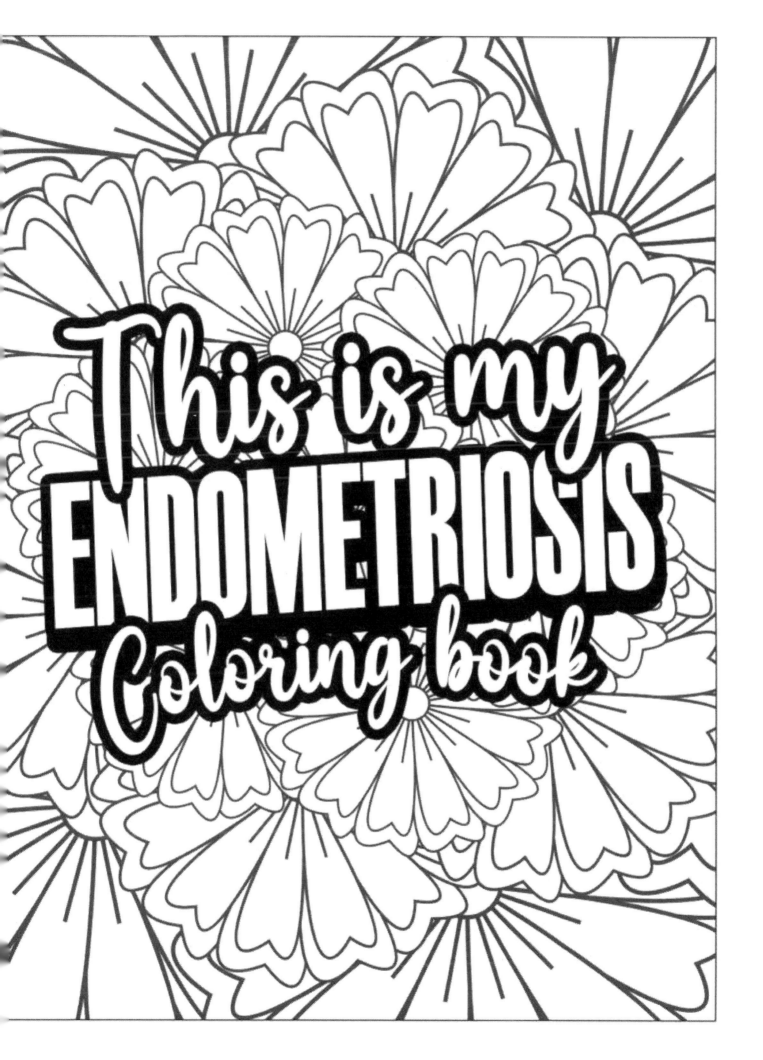

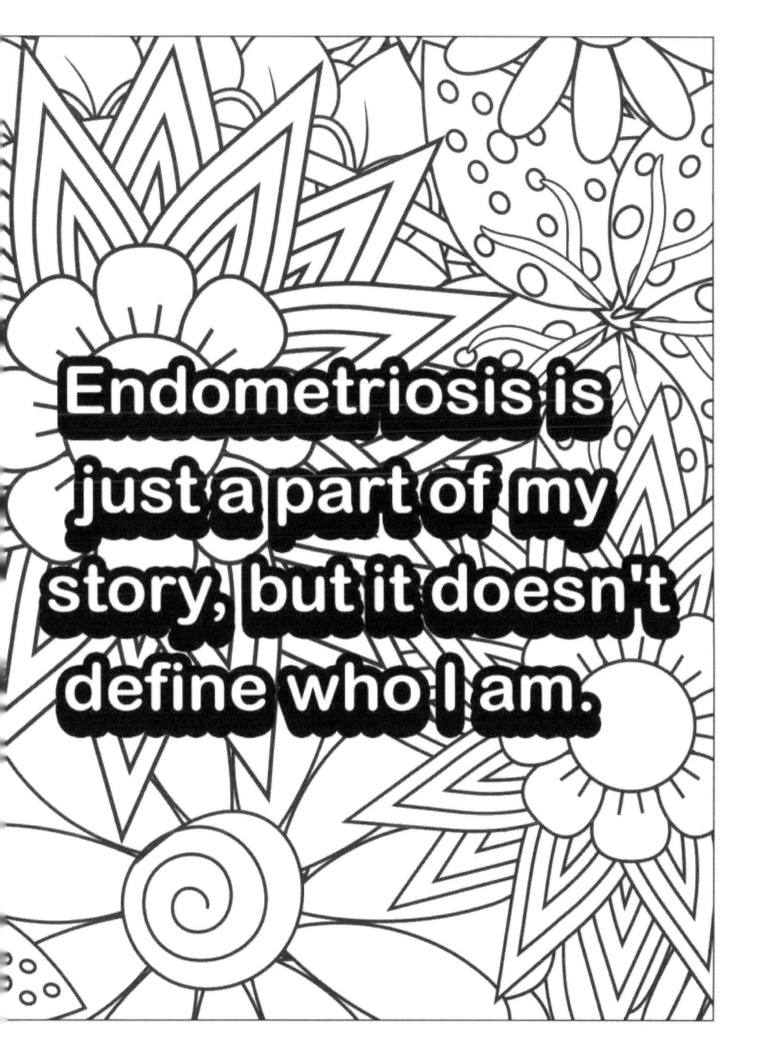

Endometriosis is just a part of my story, but it doesn't define who I am.

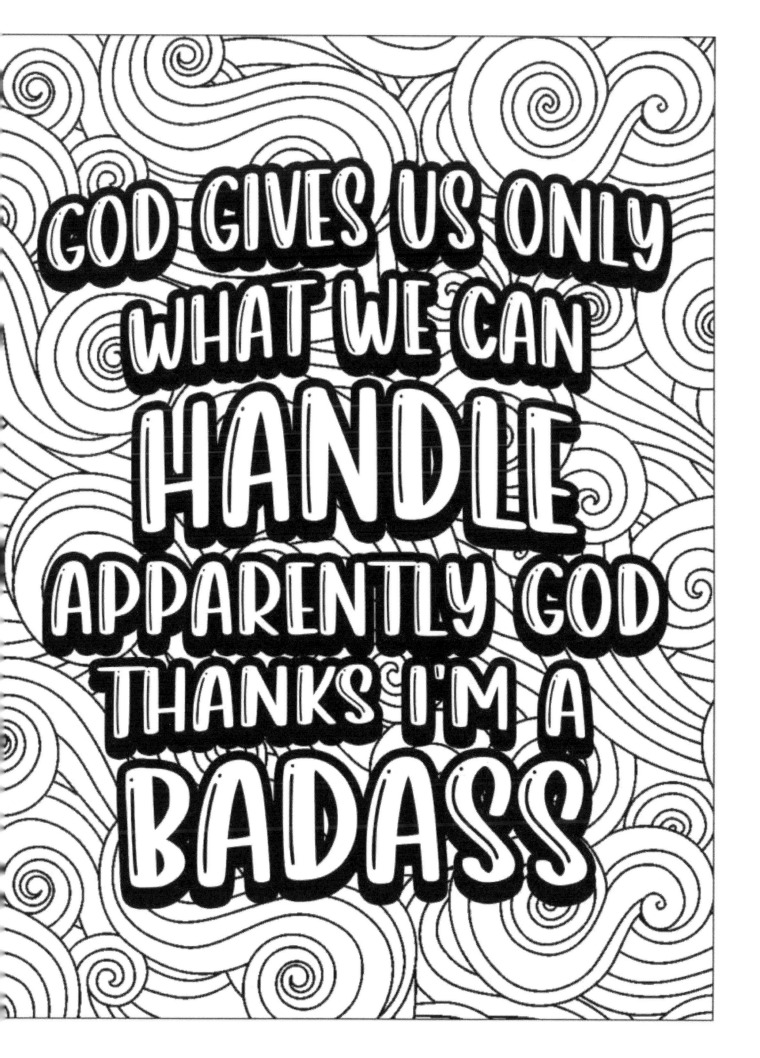

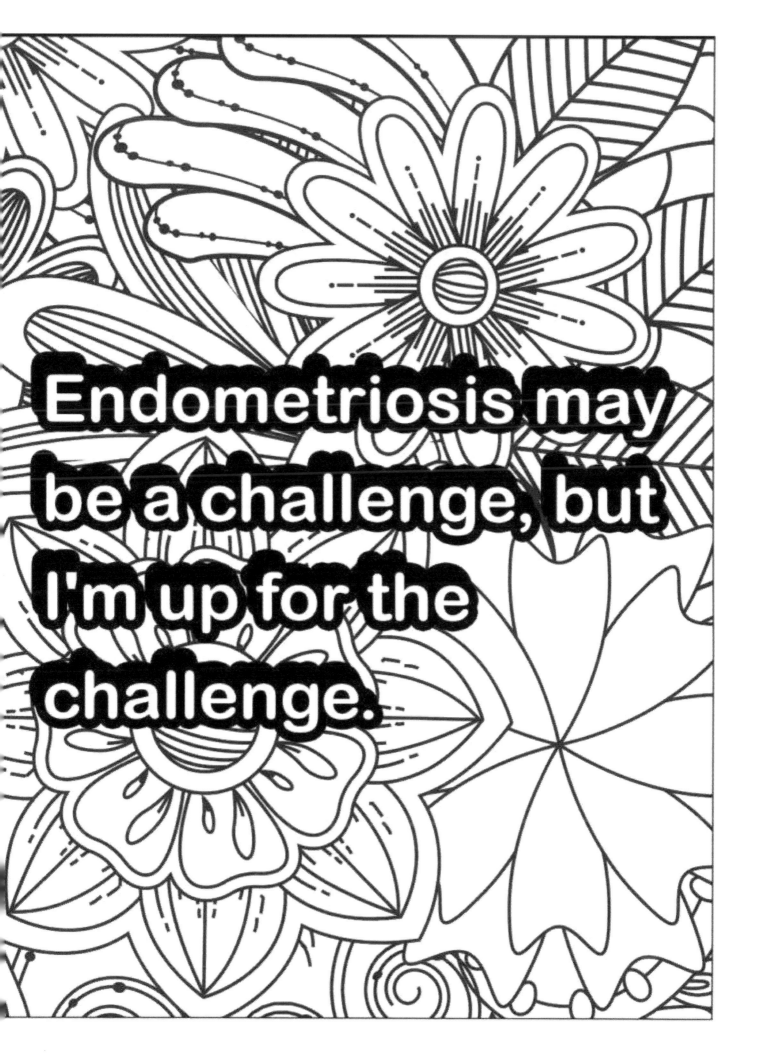

Endometriosis may be a challenge, but I'm up for the challenge.

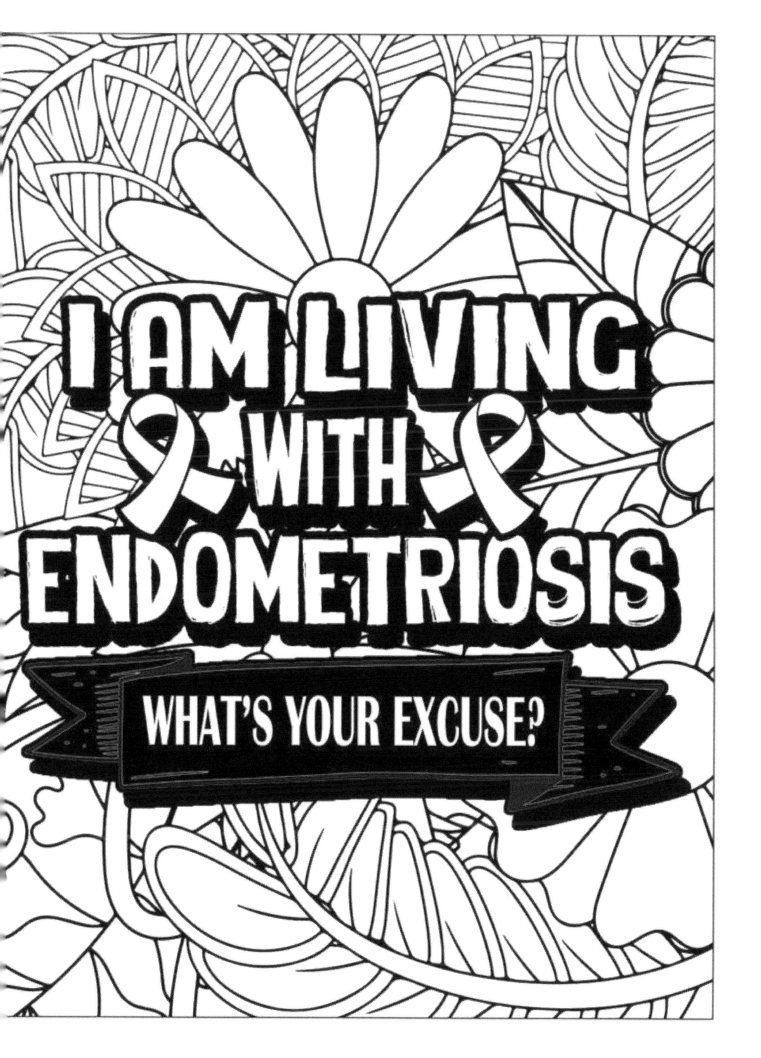

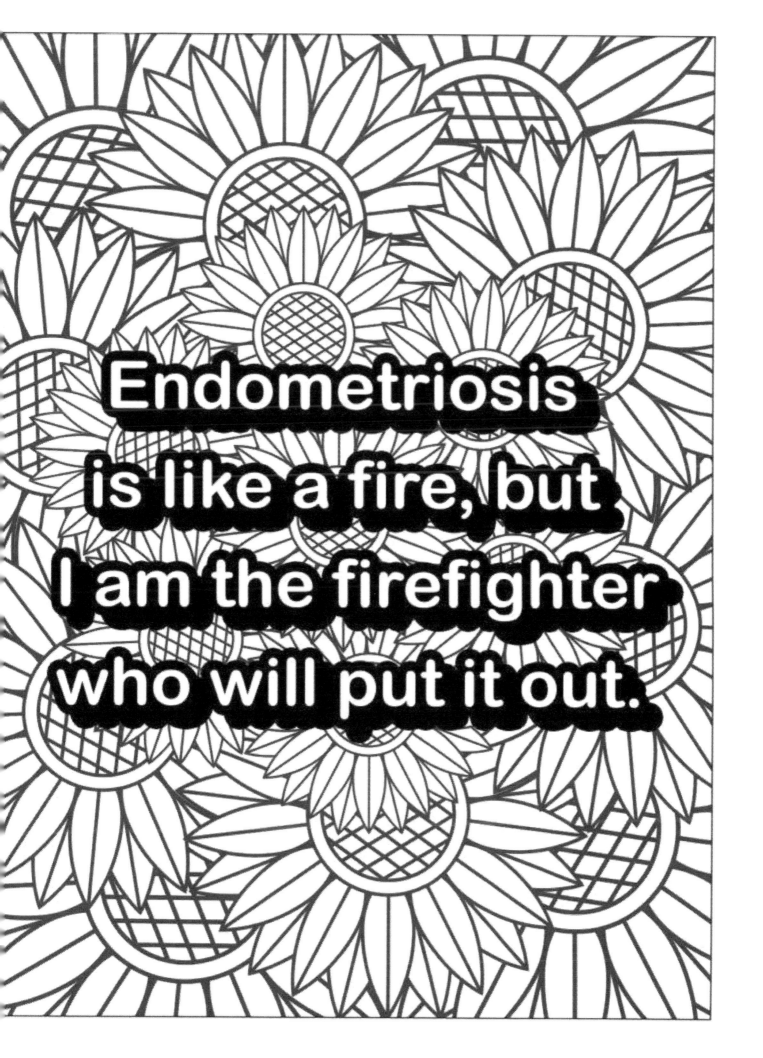

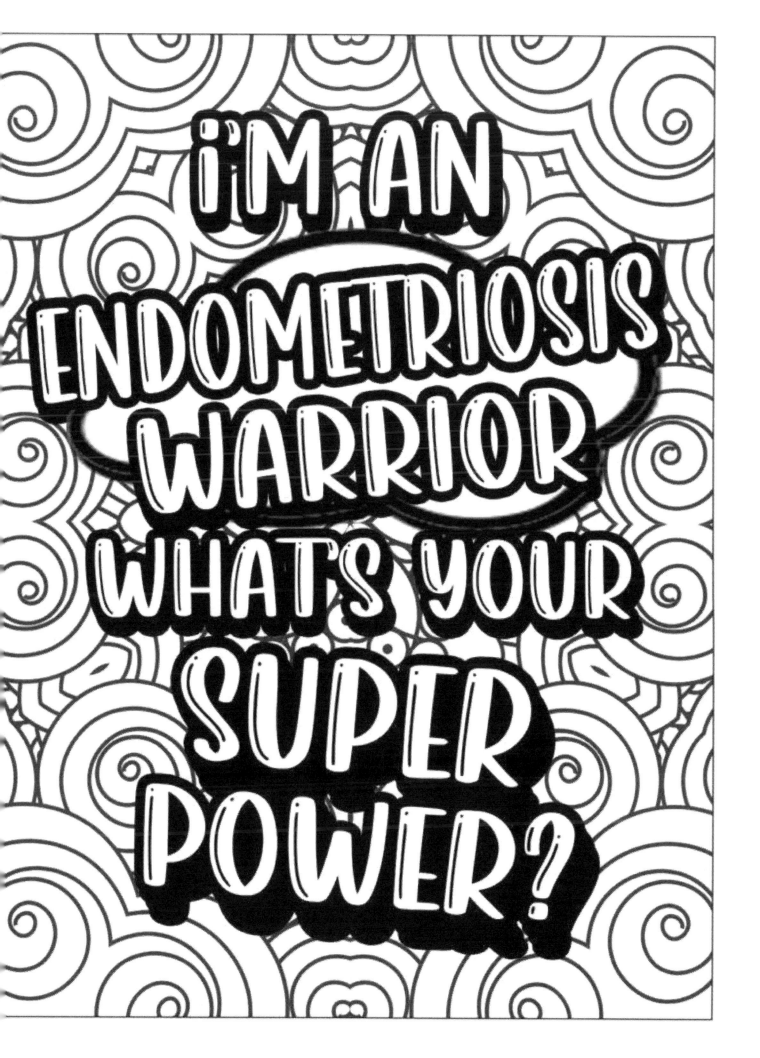

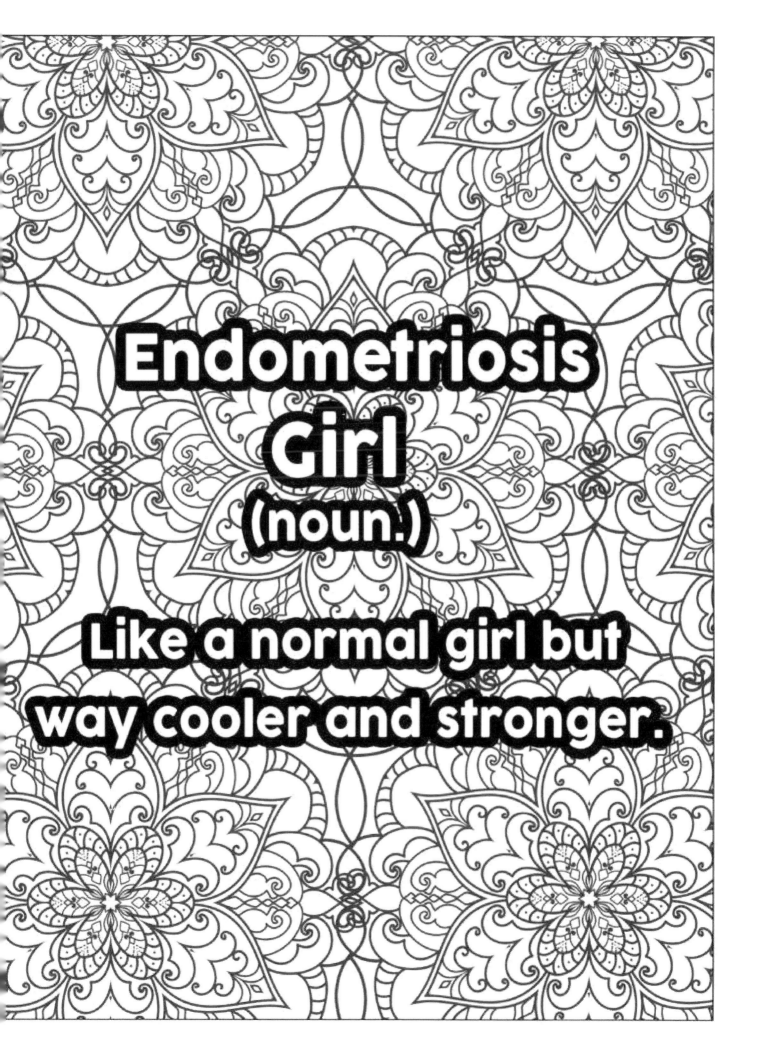

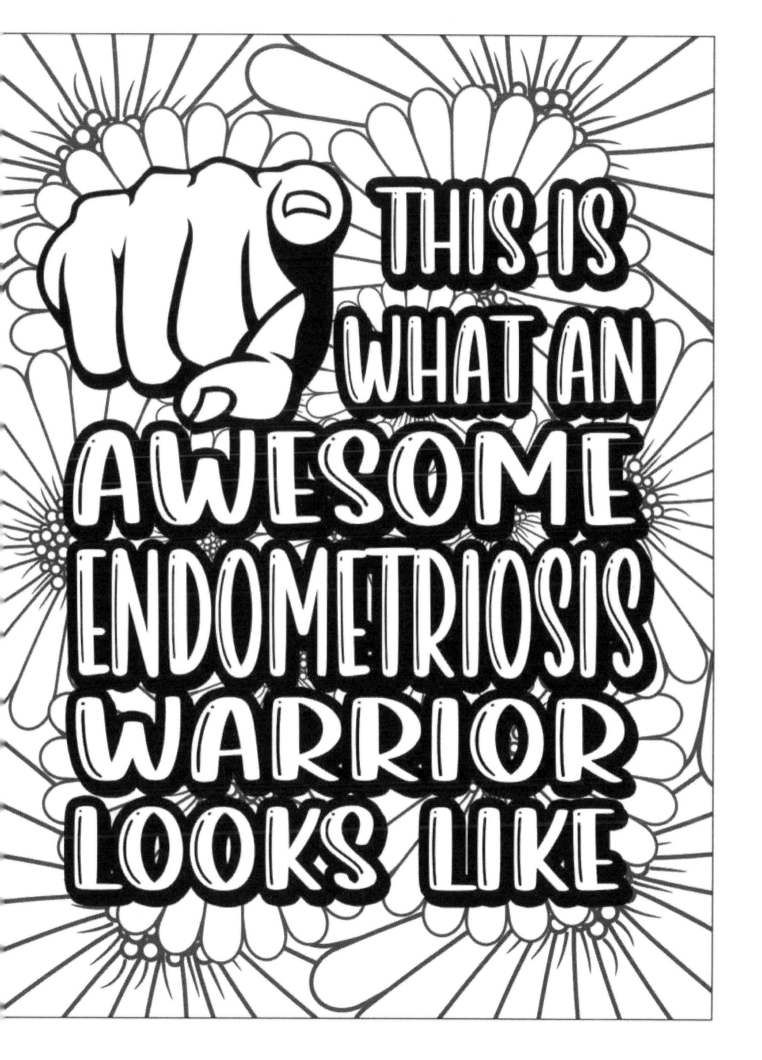

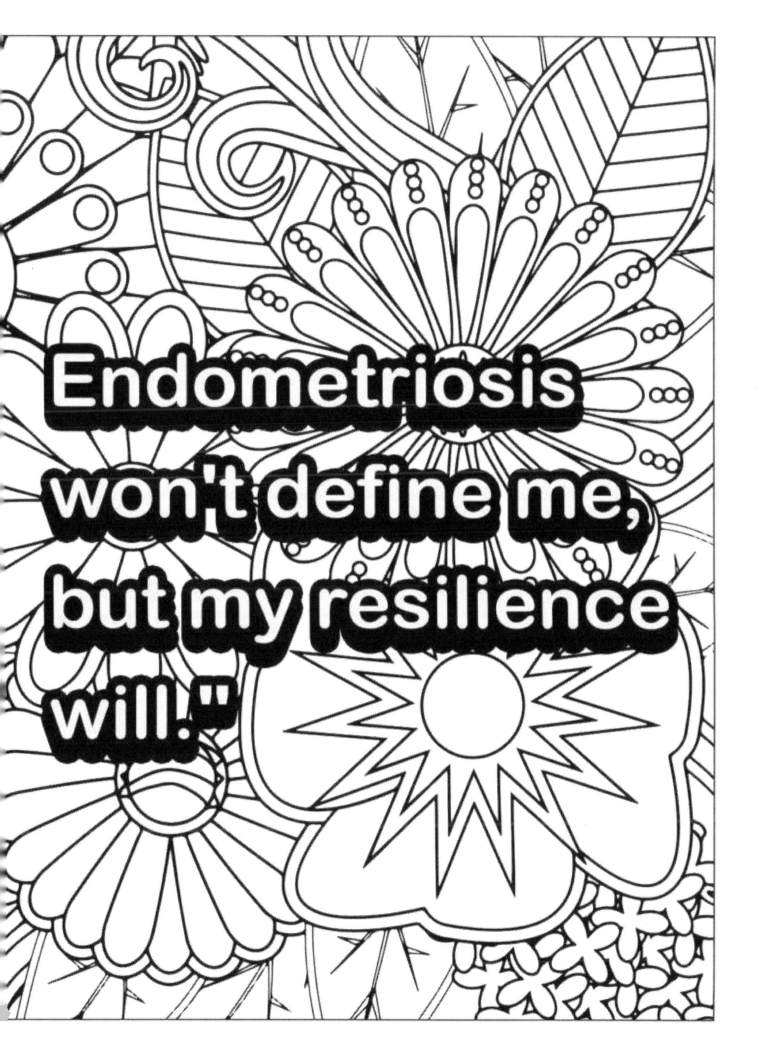

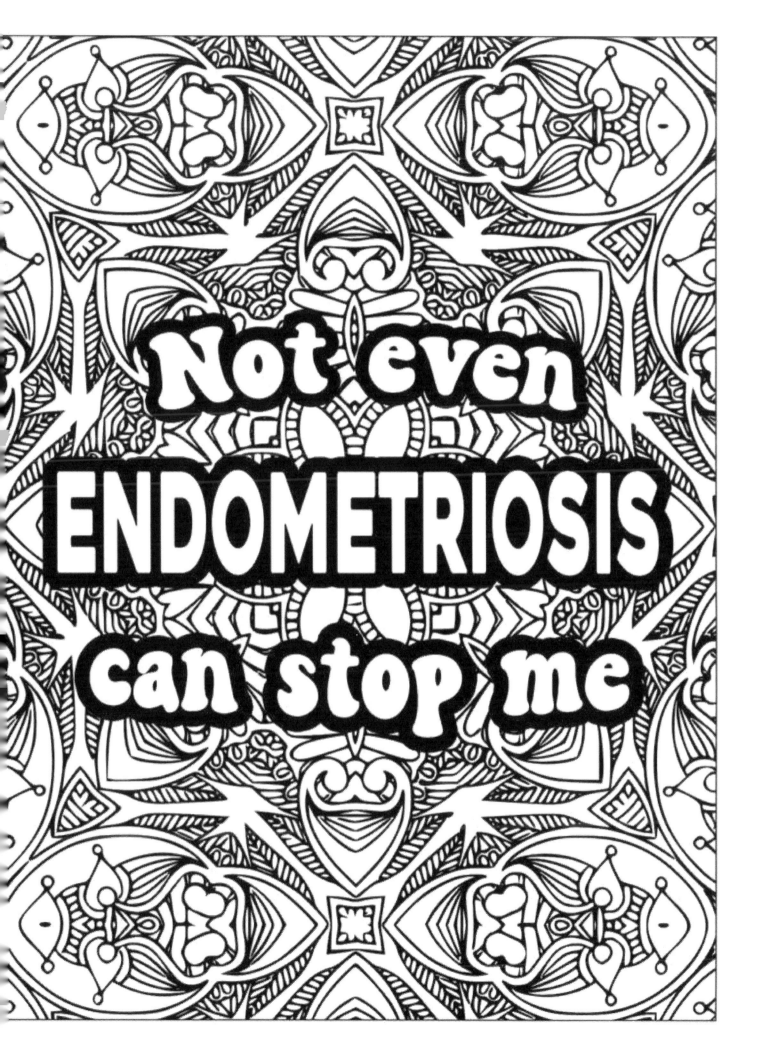

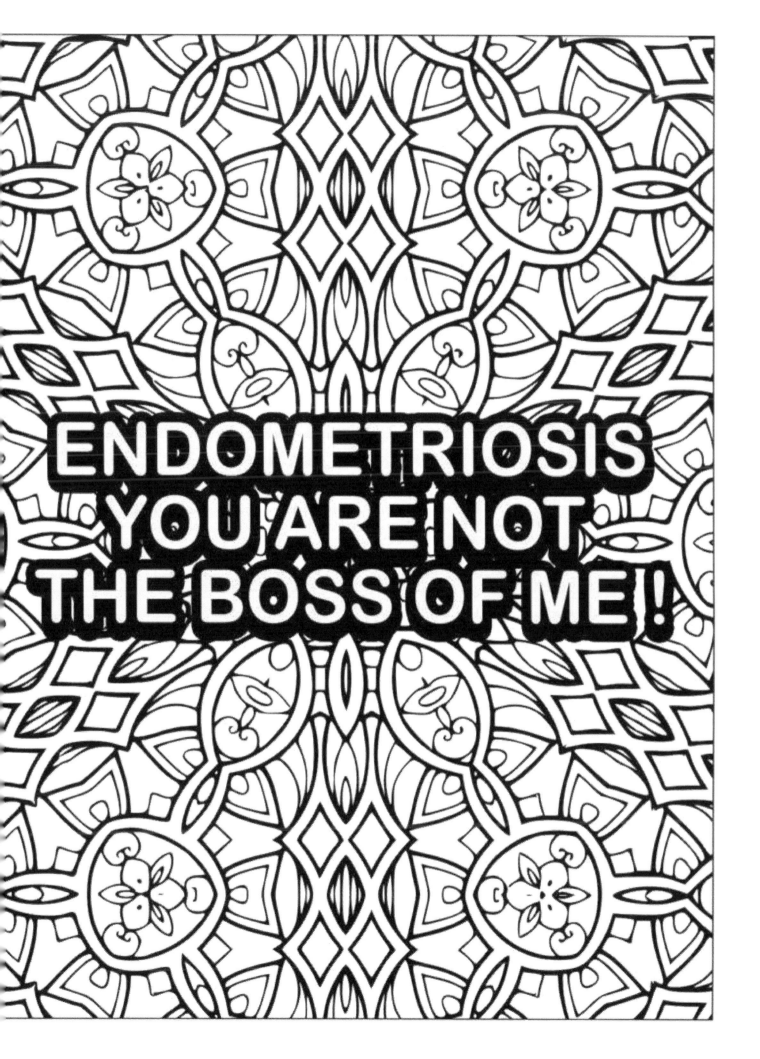

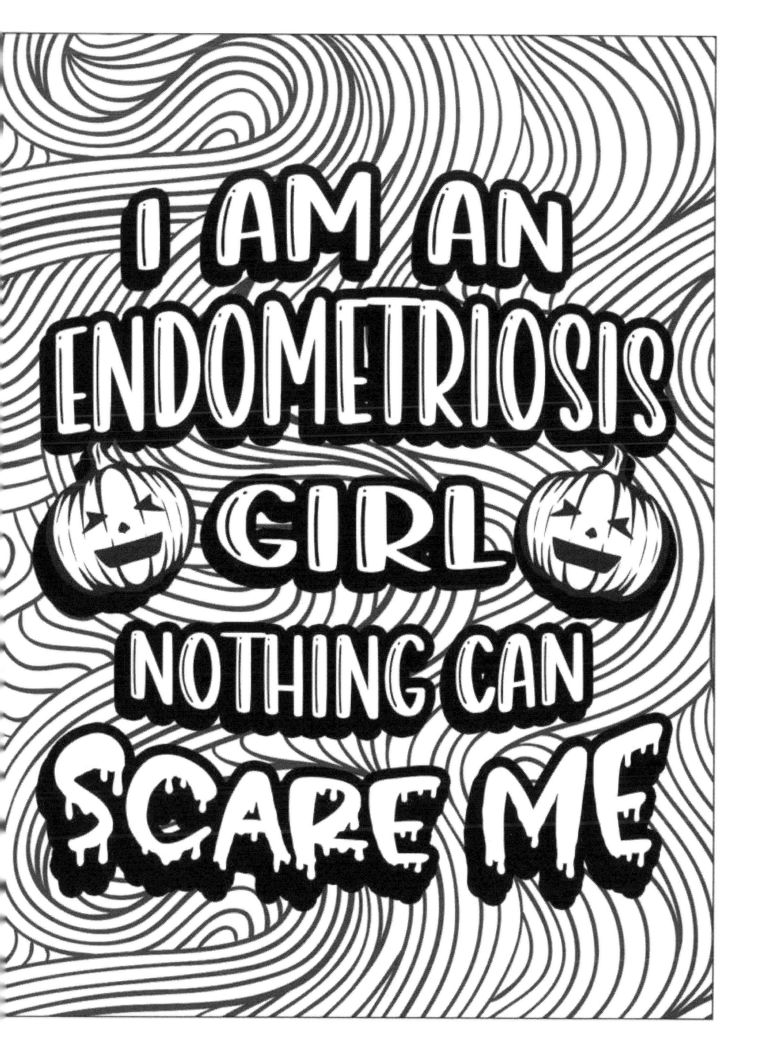

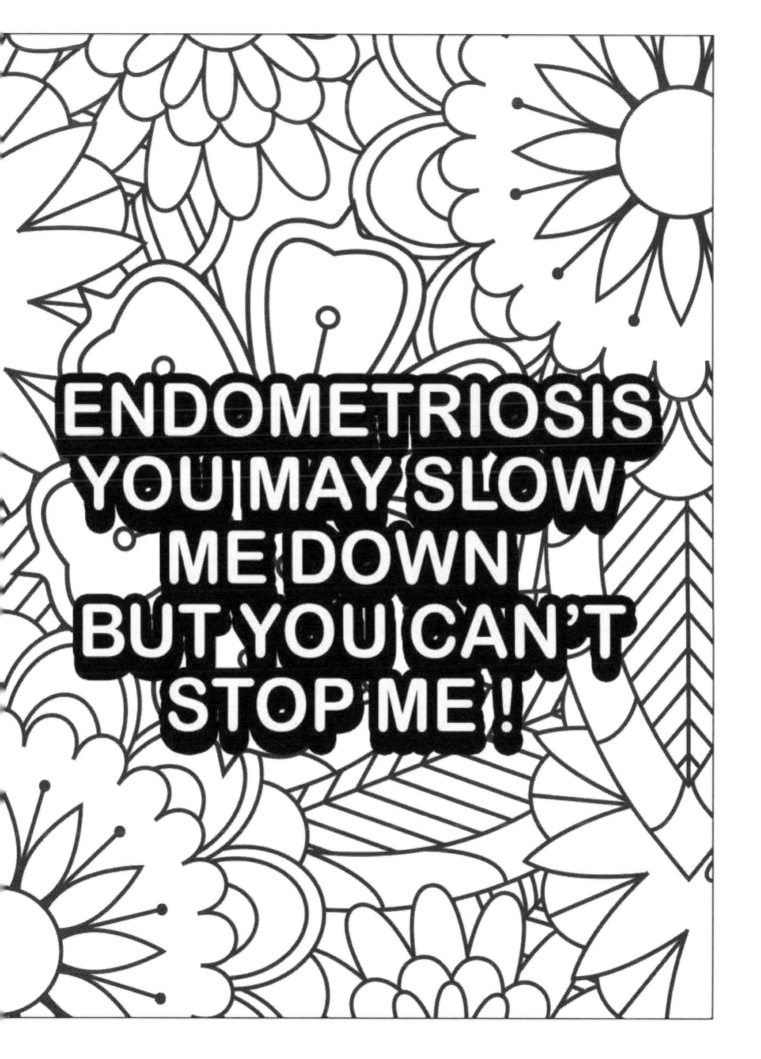

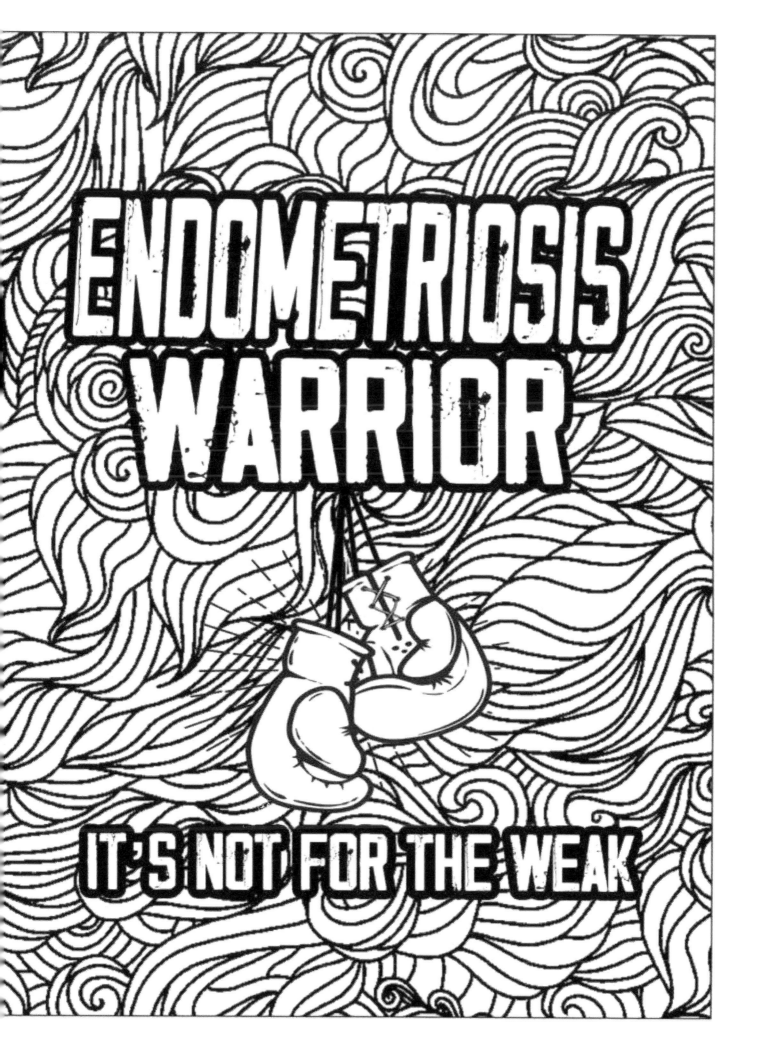

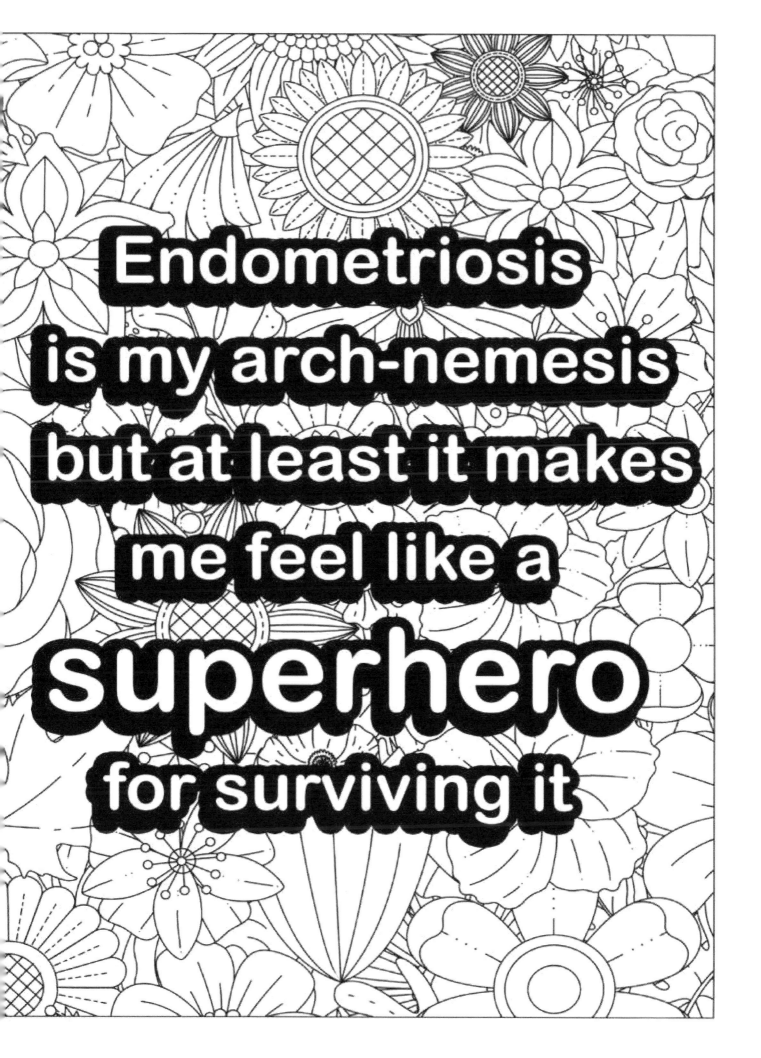

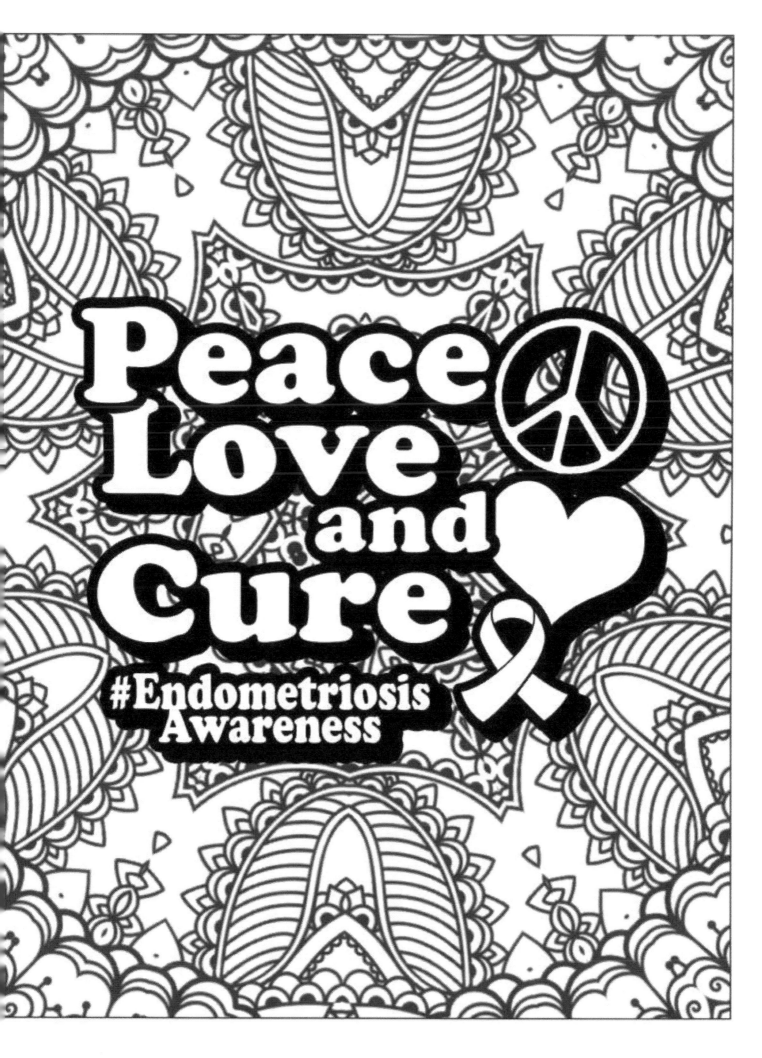

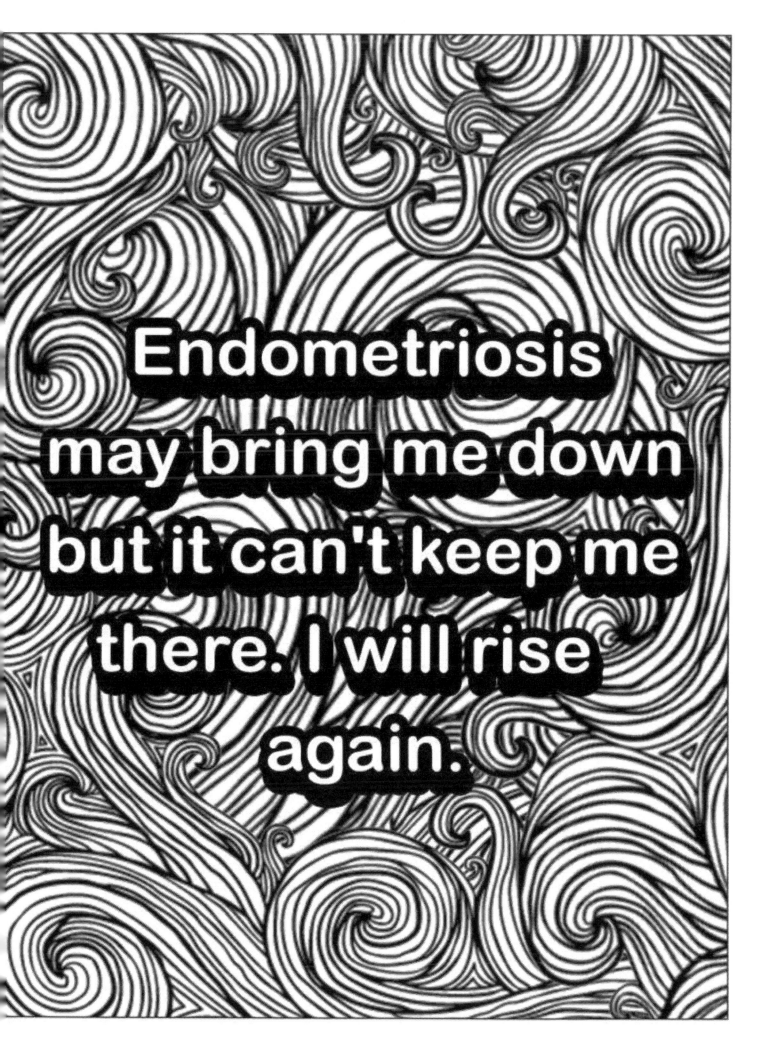

Endometriosis may bring me down but it can't keep me there. I will rise again.

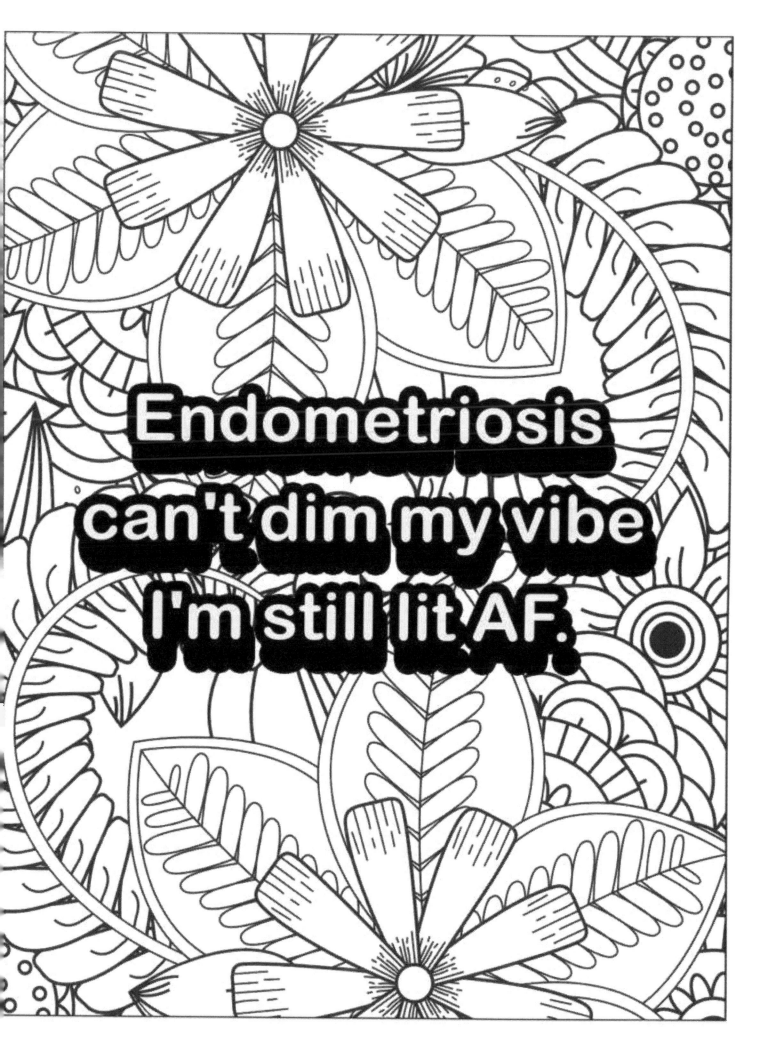

Endometriosis can't dim my vibe I'm still lit AF.

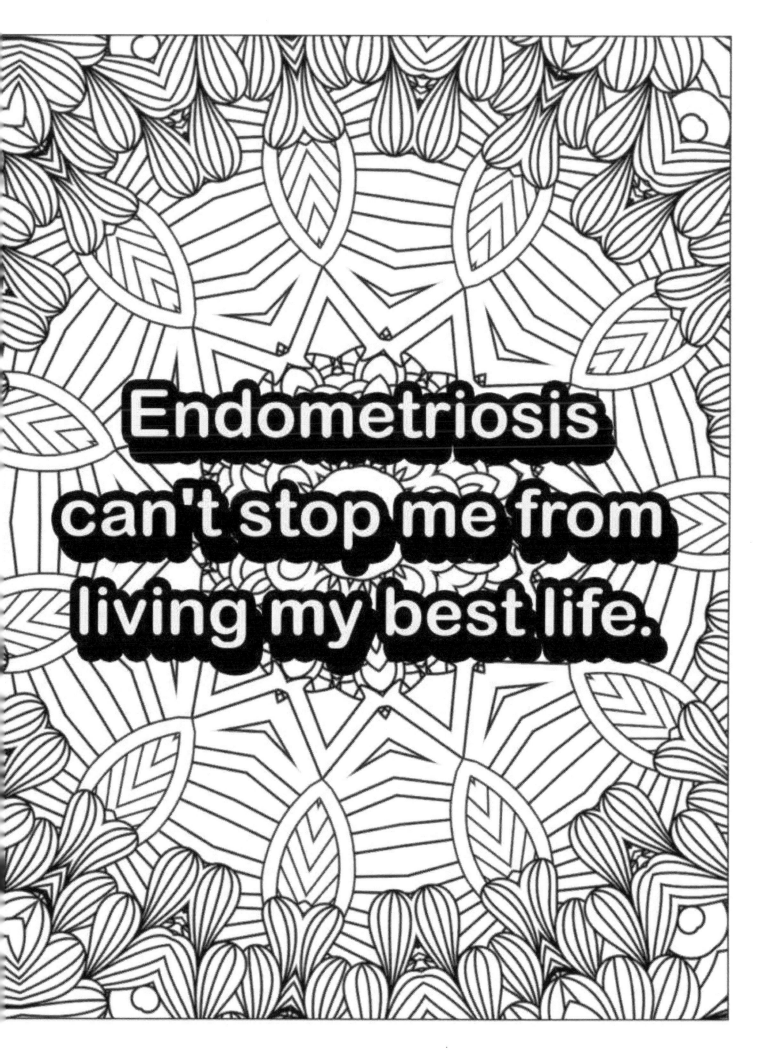

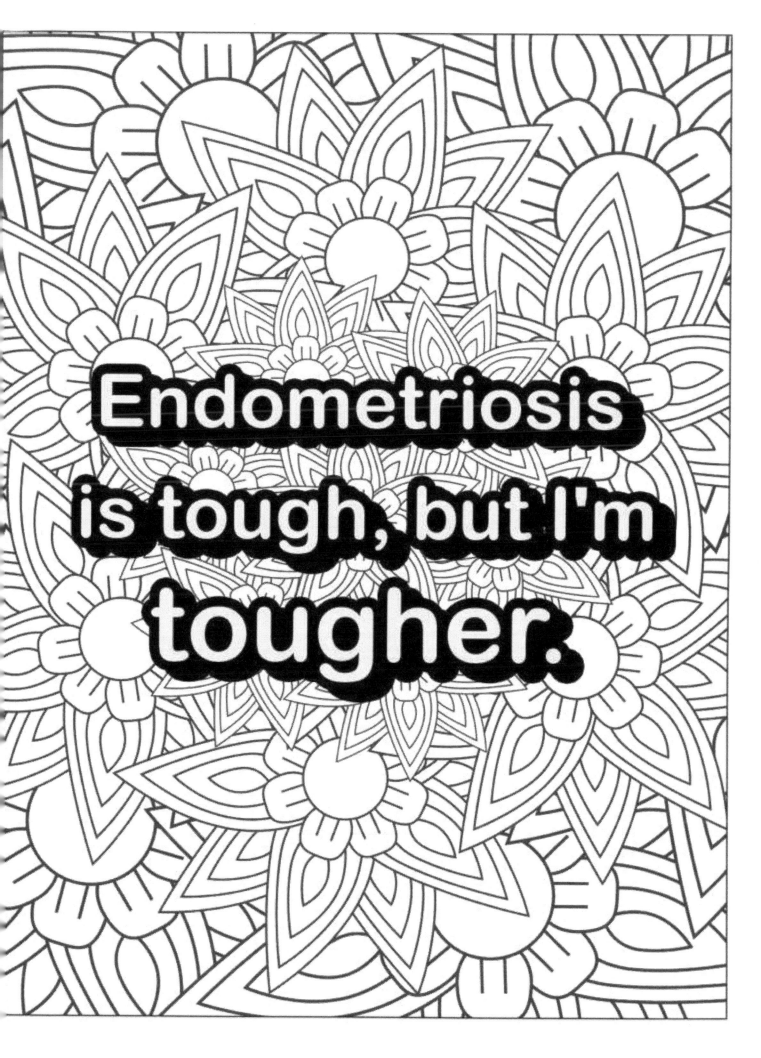

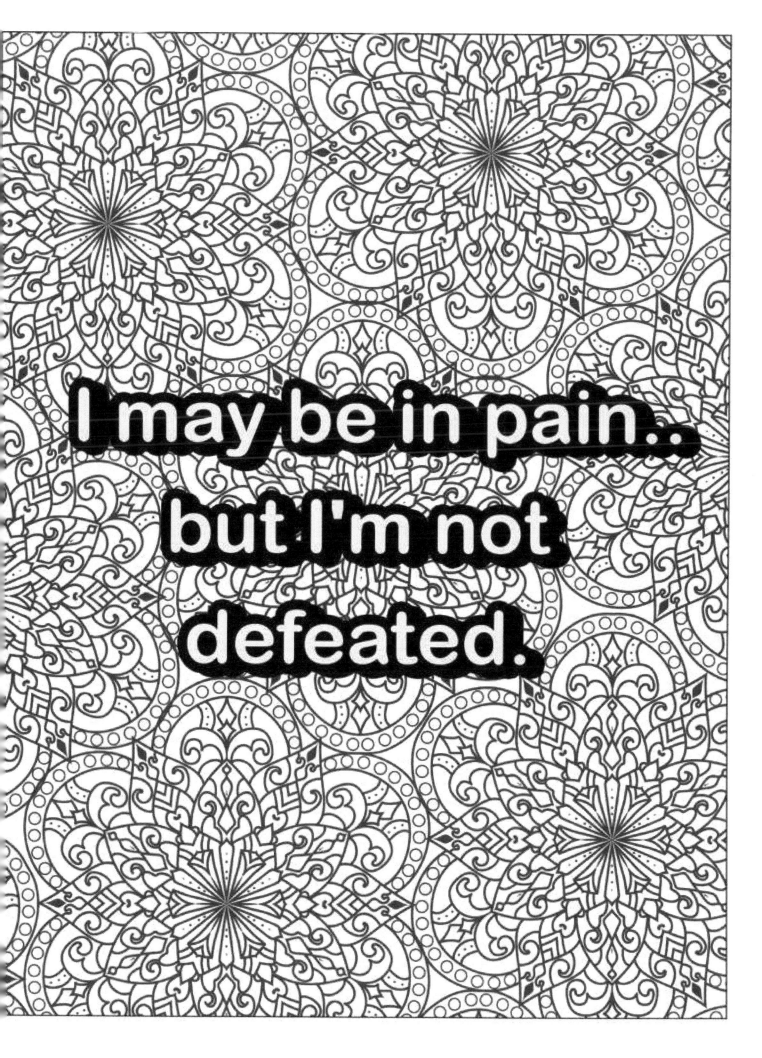

I may be in pain... but I'm not defeated.

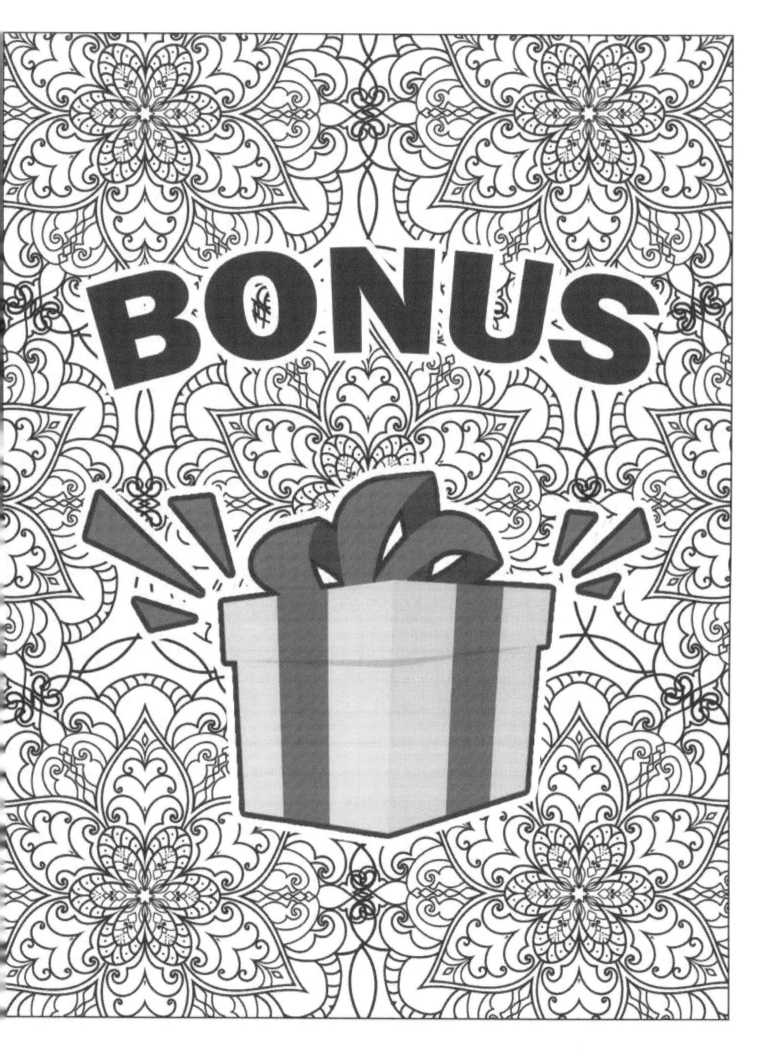

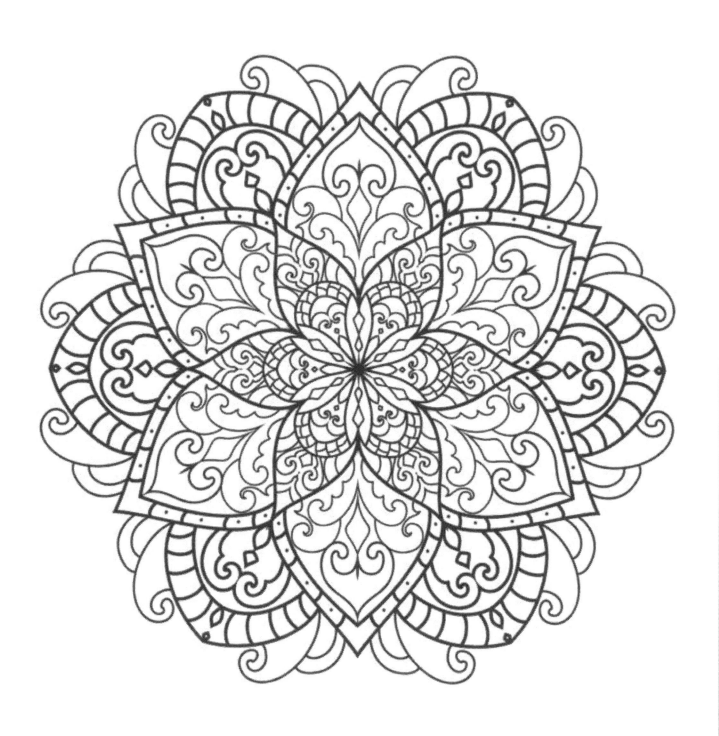

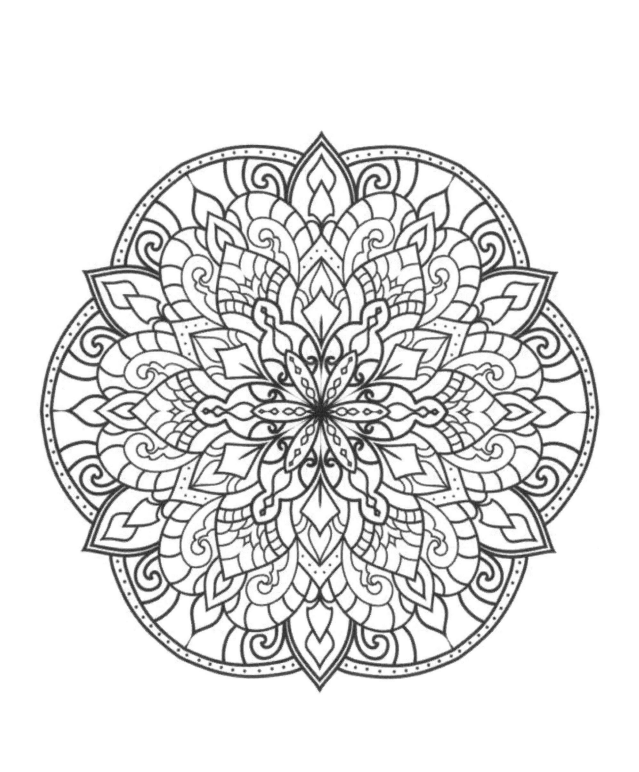

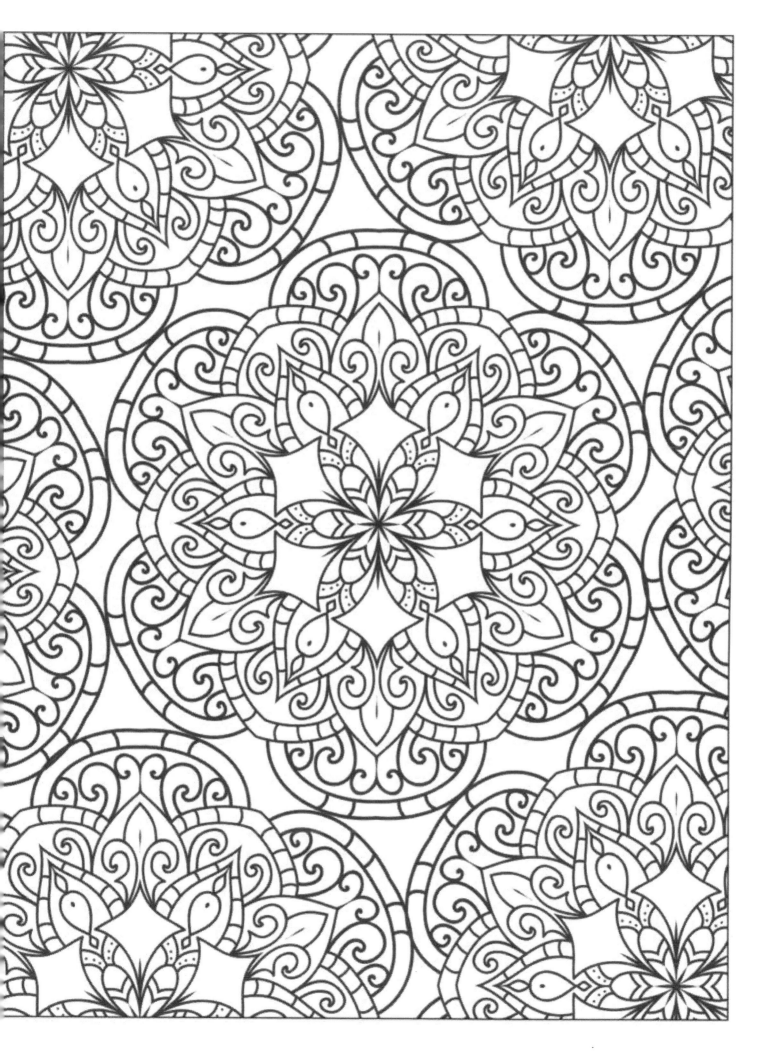

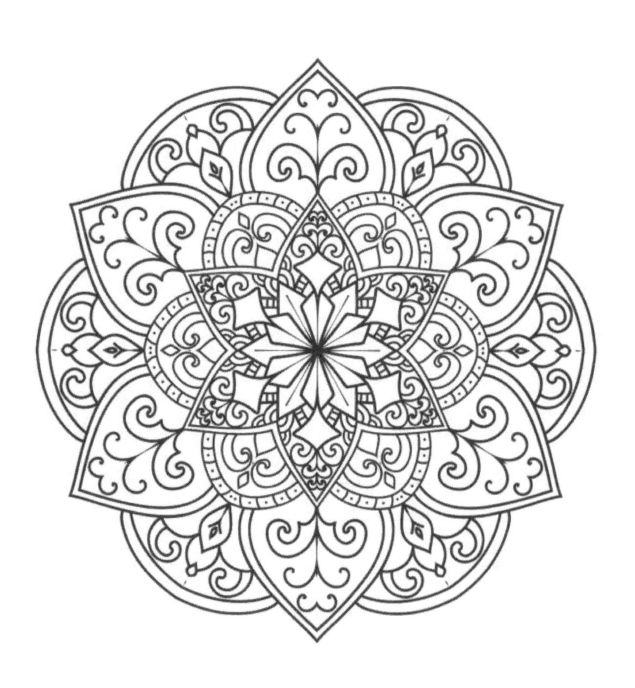

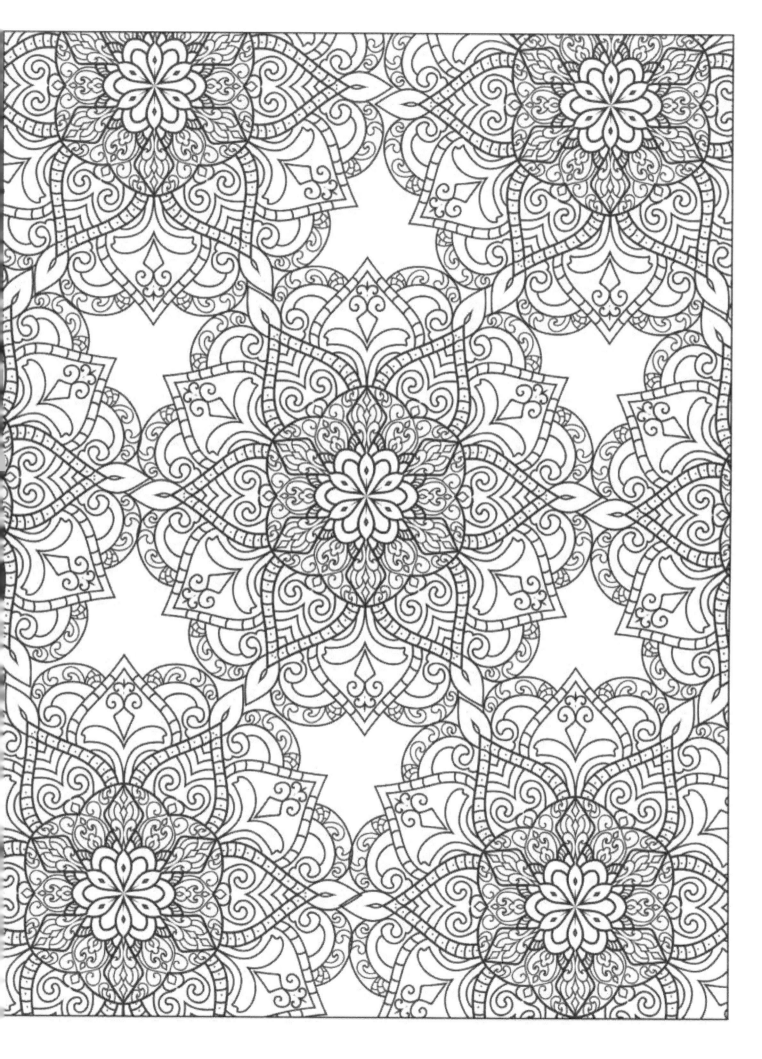

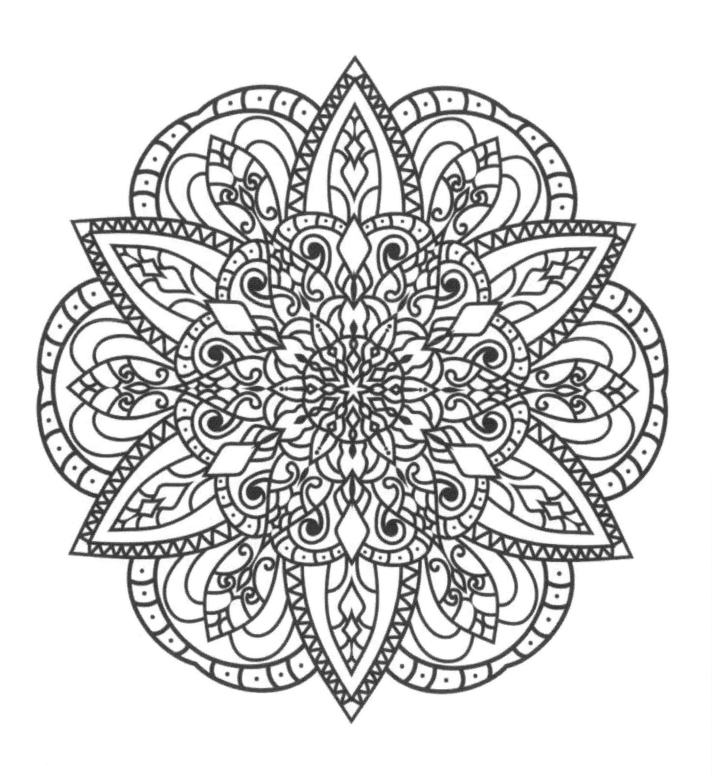

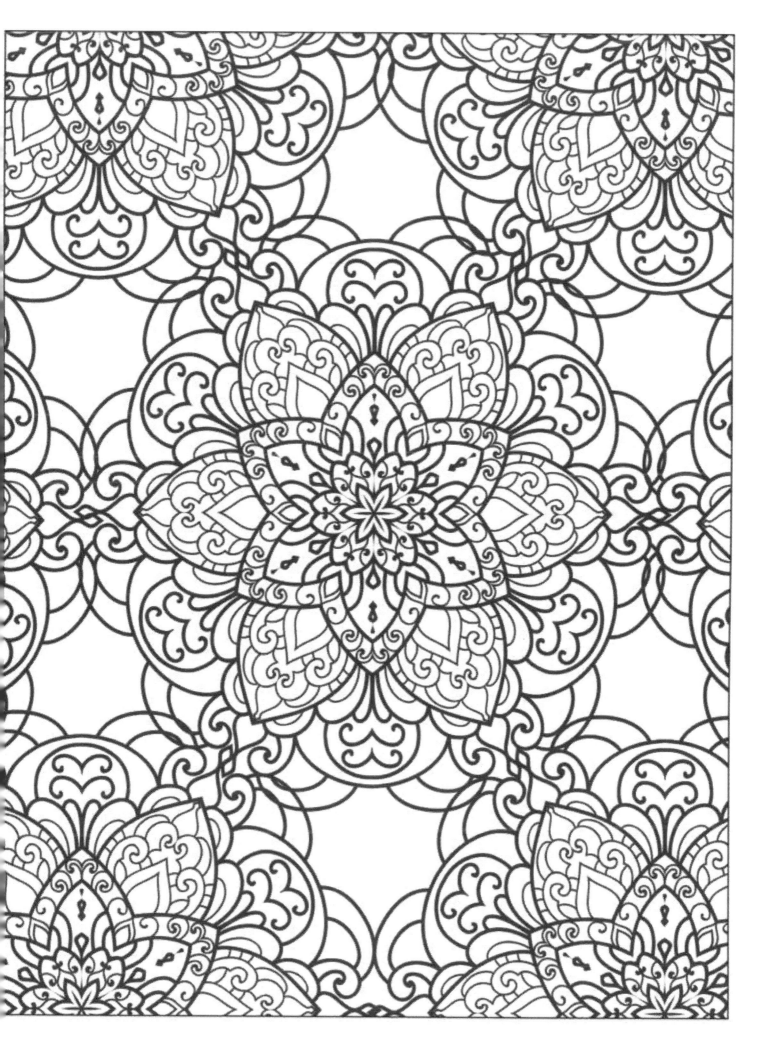

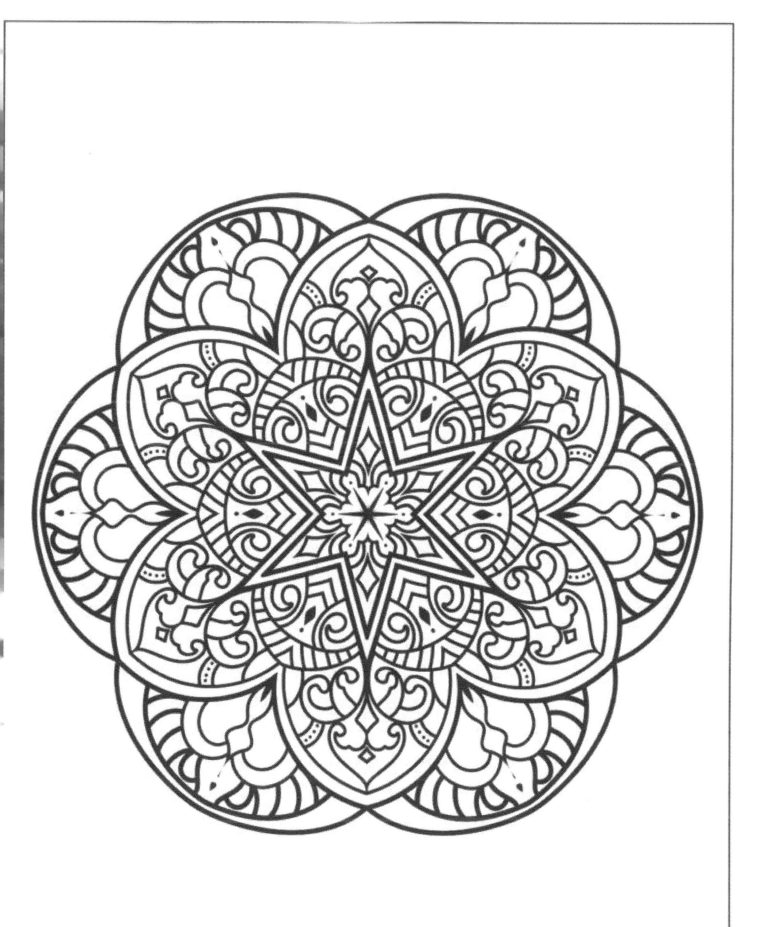

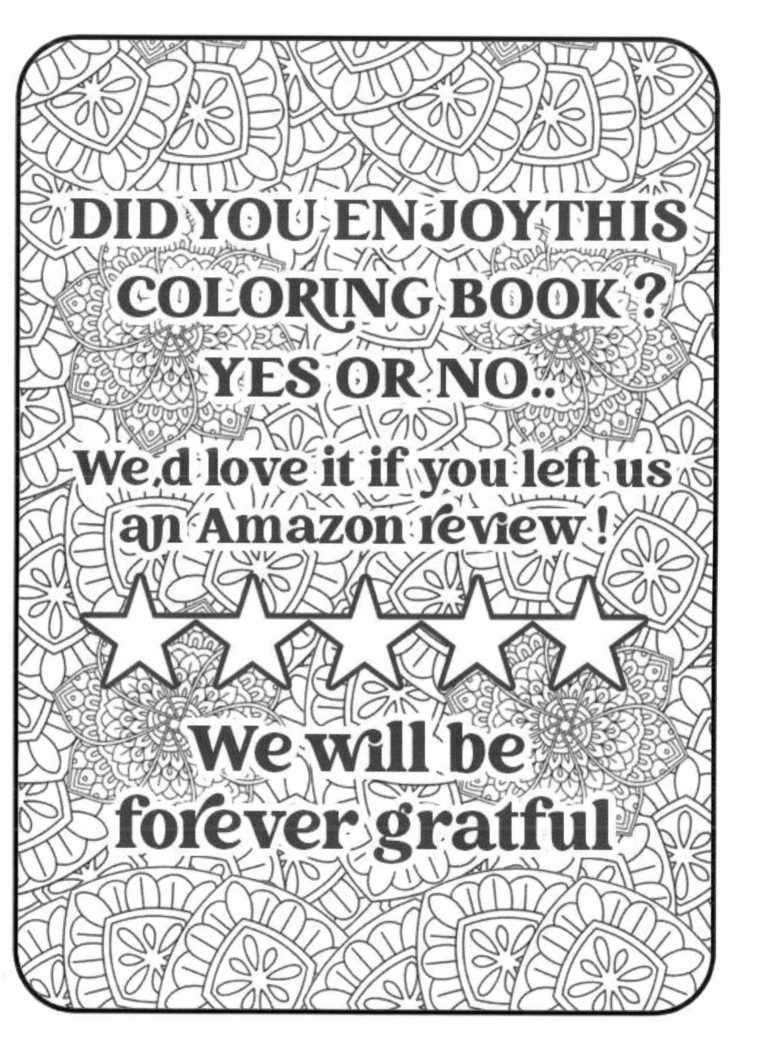

Made in the USA
Las Vegas, NV
05 October 2024

96352630R00039